Couples Sex Guide: Mastering the Intimate Massage

The Ultimate Guide to Spice up the Bedroom.
Uncover the Secrets to a Better Sex Life!

by Dominique Atkinson

Published by:

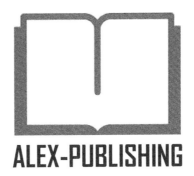

ALEX-PUBLISHING

Table of Content

Introduction 4

Massage as Foreplay 5

    Is foreplay a means to an end? 5

    Be mindful of the meaning 6

    Understand the way of Tantra 6

    Revive the ritual 7

The Technique 8

    Connect 8

    Contact 9

    Know how to use your hands 9

    Explore your lover's body 10

    Please and tease 11

    Turn over a new feel 12

    Communicate 13

Setting the Mood 14

    Peace and privacy 14

    Feather the nest 14

    It's up to you to lubricate or not 15

    Bathe or shower 15

Give Her Pleasure (Yoni Massage) 16

    Yoni massage is a form of worship 16

    Expect the extremely ecstatic 16

    Prepare to worship 17

    Position yourself for maximum pleasure 17

    Hold heaven in your hands 18

    Give her pleasure in four ways 18

    Massaging the labia 18

Massaging the clitoris 19

Massaging the vagina 19

Massaging the G-spot 20

Experiment with positions 21

Give Him Pleasure (Lingam Massage) 22

Surrender your will 22

Take the lead 22

Put him in place before you begin 23

Play with pleasure in three ways 24

Massaging the testicles 24

Massaging the penis 24

Massaging the perineum 25

End happily 25

Do's and Don'ts 27

The Importance of Communication 29

**** PREVIEW OTHER BOOKS BY THIS AUTHOR**** 30

Introduction

Have your busy lives left no room for excitement in the privacy of your bedroom when you are alone with each other? Does your lover fail to understand your need to cuddle after you make love? Do you find the intensity or frequency of your sexual desires not matching your lover's?

Whether you are newly dating someone or whether you are in a long term relationship or an otherwise happily married couple, there's nothing as simple and easy to stimulate or reinvigorate your sex life as practicing the art of intimate massage. Making love puts a lot pressure on both the man and the woman to perform. This often leads one of them to pretend that they are interested when they are not or to rebuff the other's advances.

"Not, now darling, I have a headache," or "Was it good for you?"

"Hmm, what did you say? Oh, yeah, it was good, wasn't it?"

If you haven't yet said or heard these words then dread the day you start saying or hearing them. Or stop worrying and start connecting with your lover, not just on a merely physical level but emotionally, intuitively, mentally and spiritually, as well. This book will show you how to turn not just your home but any place where you are alone with your lover into a pleasure palace minus the pressure of performance. Intimate massage is not about achieving a goal or climaxing but purely about providing pleasure to your lover. So you are not focused on reaching a goal but on creating a connection with your lover. Unlike mere foreplay where the objective is still to have sex, an intimate massage is an entirely sensual experience that involves your whole body, mind and spirit. Of course, if it naturally leads to sex, which it often does, then it's entirely up to you to choose what to do.

When you give your lover a sensual and intimate massage, you are not expecting anything in return but you are completely engrossed in giving him or her pleasure. While it helps your lover relax and enjoy the massage, it offers you the freedom and convenience to open not only your eyes, but your mind and body as well to a whole new way of experiencing intimacy.

The intimate massage is not a novelty but an ancient ritualistic practice common in Eastern traditions. In fact, in many cultures, it is a natural expression of love. As we became more materialistic and our lives got busier, nobody had the time or inclination to make love the way it should be done. After all, love is never about you as a person, is it? It is about the experience.

Give your lover an intimate massage and bring back the connection that you naturally have on a physical, sensual, spiritual and universal level.

Massage as Foreplay

An intimate massage is a great way for couples to relax and connect with each other, in more ways than you could have imagined. If you thought that a massage is all about physical contact, think again. Many a time during a massage, whether it is a full body massage, a head massage, a foot massage or any other kind, it is not uncommon for the person receiving the massage to drift off to sleep. Similarly, it is also quite normal that a person will feel refreshed and energetic after a massage. What could be the reasons for this?

It's a way to exchange energy

When we are awake, our mind is aware of what we are thinking and feeling. We are in a conscious emotional and mental state. When we relax and drift off to sleep or are in a kind of semi-drowsiness, then the mind can let go off thoughts and emotions that it is holding on to. This is why, for people who have had a busy or stressful day at work, a massage can be a powerful way to let go of the negative emotions such as worries, anger or fear.

When a person receives a massage not only are the tired muscles and joints of the body revived but the conscious mind is cleared and a person can think and feel with a clarity never felt before. When we think, exercise, run or perform any activity whether physical or mental, we expend or use energy from within our body. Similarly, when a person gives another person a massage, there is essentially an exchange of energy taking place.

This energy is not just physical but also emotional and according to some ancient Eastern traditions like Tantra, it can be sexual and spiritual as well. In fact, in many cultures it is believed that a massage can stimulate and strengthen the life-force energy or Prana or Chi (pronounced Qi) which flows not only within a person but also connects us with a universal or cosmic source of energy. Therefore a massage can reinvigorate vitality and what better or more pleasurable way to do this than through a slow, sensual and intimate massage?

Is foreplay a means to an end?

Making love begins with foreplay and ends in orgasm. Or at least this is what is considered as the conventional or normal course of action during sex. For most people, sexual intercourse actually means penetration, ejaculation, orgasm or climax. And nothing more, nothing less.

Stimulation, pleasure, intimacy, communication and sharing are all secondary. Nothing could be more far from the truth because for the act of making love to have meaning, you need to spend some time and think about it.

So even though I know you are keen to start reading about the techniques of intimate massage, I request you to please bear with me and take a few minutes to understand why and how an intimate massage can bring back the magic of making love.

Once you realize the relevance and benefits of giving and receiving an intimate massage, you will start looking at making love from a whole new perspective.

Most often during sex, the people involved are caught up in a frenzy of physical and emotional expression where most often there is very little attention paid to what is being felt or not. You may light candles and play soft music or even use toys but does the actual act of making love still feel like it's lacking in something?

Is it intensity or sensuality? Even for the most loving and most romantic couples, sex sometimes becomes an automatic or habitual encounter rather than a special or intensely enjoyable experience. Why is this so?

Be mindful of the meaning

When you watch a talented actor or musician on stage, you can witness the pleasure the person is feeling in his performance. This is the same with an artist or a sportsperson, a magician or any man or woman who does something with complete concentration and involvement in the work at hand. They are not doing it for the applause or the money, they are doing it for themselves and the pleasure that they derive from practicing their art.

Now, you may protest by saying that not all of us are artists but that some of us are just plumbers or electricians and not pianists or entertainers. Wrong. All of us are artists. No matter what work or chore it is you are doing, you can transform it and make it meaningful if you want to. In other words, if you want to you can raise any task no matter how mundane it is into an art. To do this, you have to put your heart and soul into what you are doing and be mindful of every moment while you are doing it. This is what differentiates a thespian from a ham actor, a champion from a player or a contender or a lover from a mere sexual partner. Mindfulness or being in the present and now is an important aspect of enjoying our life.

So stop being a partner, a boyfriend, a girlfriend or a spouse and start becoming a lover. Raise the act of making love into an art form and transform every moment of intimacy into a highly fulfilling experience both for you and your lover. You can just be an ordinary lover or you can become a great lover forever by mastering the art of intimate massage.

Understand the way of Tantra

When we start treating sex as just another mechanical or physical act, we spoil its sanctity or spiritual aspect. At this point, you may be wondering how sex can even be associated with something spiritual or sacred.

In one of the ancient spiritual practices from the East, known as Tantra, making love was considered an essential part of life and living, and as a means of gaining spiritual wisdom or enlightenment. While the exact meaning of Tantra is difficult to express since it is a word from a long forgotten and seldom used language, Sanskrit, it is often associated with the science of cosmic energy and the mysticism of sound and rhythm.

It involves practices or rituals that attempt to connect a person with the energy within oneself and the energy which is available all around us in the universe, and also to find that perfect rhythm or balance with which everything makes sense or which brings meaning to our existence. If this sounds obtuse and is difficult to comprehend, do not despair. Tantra isn't supposed to be understood but experienced. Most of the Tantric principles are concerned with expanding our consciousness and understanding of life through meditation and rituals.

Revive the ritual

Almost any kind of massage has a ritualistic as well as a meditative aspect to it just as it combines physical movements with mindfulness. To practice the art of intimate massage, you need to be aware of both the mindful or meditative aspect and the ritualistic.

It is therefore important that you regularly spend some time contemplating about or thinking about your lover and your relationship. This is, in some ways, a form of meditation. While popular perception of meditation forms the image of sitting cross legged in silence or chanting or humming a mantra, it's not exactly correct. Meditation is simply spending some quality time alone with your own self or a kindred spirit or spirits.

You can meditate alone or meditate with your lover and you will see demonstrated later in this book how you can combine meditation and massage so that it becomes an enjoyable and enlightening experience for both of you, physically and emotionally, stimulating and relaxing at the same time.

Making love is a form of ritual. The integral part of a ritual is that it consists of a series of activities or actions that are performed in a specific order. Consider some everyday rituals like making tea or coffee or tying your shoelace or necktie.

To make coffee, you first put the coffee powder in a cup and then pour hot water, isn't it? Now instead, how about pouring hot water and then adding the coffee? Or how about pouring cold water and then boiling the water and coffee together? Similarly, when you are tying a shoe lace or a necktie, there are certain knots that you make out of habit. Instead of doing it the usual way, how about if you do it a different way? It wouldn't come out right, would it? Neither will the coffee taste right nor will the necktie look right or feel comfortable.

You can't take short cuts or change the order of a ritual. Making love is similar. Foreplay is essential. In our busy daily routines, we have compressed traditional rituals and come up with concepts like instant coffee or readymade ties. We tried to do the same with making love and we have corrupted sex. We've made it a means to an end. We've cut short the process. We go fast when we should go slow.

The "Art of the Intimate Massage" revives the ritual of foreplay in lovemaking as it used to be and should be. Slow, sensual and satisfying for both people involved.

The Technique

If you want to learn how to become a great lover, then it is essential to learn how to connect, make contact and communicate with your lover. Connect, contact and communicate — these are the three key stages involved in the technique of giving and receiving an intimate massage.

Before we examine the different stages, it is important to note and remember that you are committed to spend some time (at least an hour) to do an intimate massage. Why? That's because the intimate massage described in this chapter is a full body massage and anything less than an hour would not give the receiver sufficient time to relax or enjoy the massage. Also note that while the main intention is to provide pleasure to the receiver, it is also meant to help him or her relax. So you should mutually agree to define what is within or off limits.

Until you fully complete the full body massage sequence described herein, it is advised that you refrain from any specific sexual stimulation. In other words do not focus or linger on your lover's sex centers such as the female vagina and clitoris or the male genitals and penis even though you may be tempted to indulge in it because it can cut short the full body massage.

After all, the objective of the full body intimate massage is to please and perhaps tease but not to engage in sex or achieve an orgasm. The ideal time to massage your lover's sex centers would be following a full body massage because it will heighten their pleasure. You will be delighted to know that are two separate chapters each dedicated to massaging the female sex center including massage techniques to stimulate the vagina, the clitoris and the G-spot and the male genitals and penis.

Connect

Before you begin the massage session, make sure you are on the same wavelength as your lover. How to do this? Start by standing or sitting down on the floor, facing each other. You can place a mat or a mattress on the floor if that makes you more comfortable. Ideally, both of you should have undressed and are completely naked. However, if you wish to you can use this preliminary stage before starting the massage to undress each other. It is recommended that both you and your lover bathe or take a shower before the massage session.

You may hold hands or stay apart without touching each other. Again, this is a matter of choice and comfort levels. Gaze at your lover and look deep into his or her eyes. Do you feel odd or embarrassed to do this? Then it makes it all the more important why you should do this because you may have forgotten how to connect with your lover.

There is no need to speak if you don't want to but feel free to say something or whisper it softly in your lover's ear if you wish to do so. The important thing is to make eye contact, gain your lover's trust and make sure they are comfortable right in the beginning. This is important because during most of the massage session which typically should last at least an hour, your lover will be either lying face down facing away from you or lying with his or her eyes closed, in a completely relaxed state. So before you start giving an intimate massage, make that connection which binds you to each other for the rest of the session.

If you have attended an interview or made a public speech or went for a training course in public speaking, you will recognize the important role of making this connection in the beginning with your audience through eye contact. Do not rush into the next stage of physical contact. Sit facing each other comfortably for a while.

If you can sit crossed-legged in the popular meditation position commonly known as the lotus position in yoga, then do so. If you wish to you can put a cushion to sit on and be more comfortable.

Or you can kneel in front of each other or sit down on your haunches while kneeling with your feet on either side or to one side. In case you find either of these positions or any other seated position on the floor uncomfortable, then sit down on chairs facing each other.

Stay like this for as long as you feel good or want to or till you feel that you are fully relaxed and ready to go on to the next stage. It is important to understand why you are doing this before you begin the actual massage. You are essentially trying to establish that connection that exists between two people who are in love and therefore understand each other.

As the old saying goes, you know you are with someone you love when you know that you don't have to say anything to each other and when silences no matter how long they are, are never uncomfortable.

Contact

Once both of you are ready to make contact or move on to the next stage or the actual intimate massage session, have your lover lie face down comfortably on a mat or mattress on the floor. It is important to make sure the receiver of the massage is completely comfortable because he or she is going to be spending a long time, preferably an hour or more receiving an intimate and sensual massage.

If you wish to use a table such as one you may have seen in a professional massage parlor or spa, do so. If you find it comfortable and wish to do the massage while your lover is lying on the bed, you may do so provided you take the necessary precautions to cover your bed and avoid spilling any oil or lubricant you may be using. However, please note that the bed does not provide an ideal base for a massage because it does not offer an even-levelled and firm or solid support to the body when you apply pressure which is inevitable during massage.

This is the main reason why performing a massage while the receiver is lying in bed is generally not recommended because the receiver of the massage may feel uncomfortable and not be able to enjoy or gain all the benefits of the massage.

Know how to use your hands

Before we begin the sequence of the massage, let's take a few moments to become familiar with the different methods of applying pressure or giving a massage. There are seven fundamental massage techniques or methods which you may use according to both your comfort levels during the intimate massage session. These are: stroking, kneading, tapping, rubbing, caressing, pinching and pulling.

You may use some or all of these techniques while giving an intimate massage. The choice is up to both of you as the giver and the receiver to explore, experiment and to agree upon. It is therefore essential to communicate and ask for and give feedback to ensure that there is no pain or discomfort while using any technique that can make the massage unenjoyable.

Let's examine each of these techniques.

Stroking: This involves using the fingers of your hand including your thumbs to makes long or short strokes, in a gentle yet firm manner.

Kneading: Use the entire palm of your hand to apply pressure by squeezing and pressing down on the flesh gently yet firmly similar to kneading dough.

Tapping: Use the bottom edge of your palm or the edge away from your thumbs sideways to tap gently. It's similar to what you may have seen in a Karate chop but with less force.

Rubbing: Use the flat of your palm to apply even pressure in a straight or circular motion.

Caressing: This is similar to rubbing but more gently with less friction or contact between the receiver's skin and your palm.

Pinching: Take the skin and flesh between your thumb and forefinger or between the knuckles of your forefinger and middle finger and gently tug towards you.

Pulling: Take a finger, toe or a limb and pull to elongate and stretch the muscles and joints.

Explore your lover's body

Let's describe the sequence in which you can apply massage. Keep in mind that this is more than just an opportunity to physically explore your lover's body. It is an opportunity to become intimate with your lover and know how they respond to being touched in different ways and in the different parts of their body.

If you pay careful attention, it is possible to learn something new during each massage session and thereby get better at giving an intimate massage. There are not many other ways guaranteed to please your lover more. The ideal position for the giver of the massage is to kneel at the feet of the receiver if he or she is lying on the floor or stand near their feet if they are lying on a table.

Start your massage by applying the different massage techniques described earlier on your lover's feet. You may do one foot first and then the other. Do not forget to explore each toe and the space between them. Since there are many nerve endings underfoot, it is highly sensitive to touch and the receiver may feel ticklish to begin with but as the massage gradually progresses, you will sense the receiver relaxing and enjoying it. Next, massage the back of the legs, the calves and the thighs.

Start with slow, long and gentle movements and then quicken the pace, increase the intensity and pressure gradually. Taper off the pace and pressure gradually and end by being as gentle as you began.

Remember to be mindful and focus on your actions. Also keep your pace unhurried and take your time with each movement and each leg.

Please and tease

Next massage their buttocks. This is not only a very soft and sensitive part of the body but also an erogenous zone and it will do good to spend some time and effort in exploring the different ways you can pleasure your lover. It is important to note that you should focus on the massage and not indulge in any overt sexual stimulation.

Remember that while your intention is to provide pleasure, it is also important to help your lover relax. Do not abandon the massage to indulge in sex or give in to either your or your lover's need to have sex. You may tease as long as you please but control the urge to have sex.

Next, you can move on to your lover's lower back. During this stage, you may need to straddle the receiver by putting your knees on both sides of the receiver's hips. You may sit down on their buttocks while massaging the lower back but seek your lover's consent to do so. Also make sure that your weight does not hurt your lover or make him or her uncomfortable.

After this, start showering your attention and affection on the upper back and shoulders. At this point, if you find it difficult to reach then get up and kneel down on the floor facing the receiver's head so you have better access to the shoulders. Following this, sit down beside your lover first on the left and then on the right side, and slowly massage each arm, elbow, forearm, hand, palm and every finger on each hand, individually.

Resume your position in front of your lover's head and massage their neck and head. This is a rare and wonderful opportunity for you to gently explore the erogenous zones around your lover's neck as well as around and behind the ears.

In the beginning we mentioned the different ways to use your hands to perform the massage. There are a few variations you may try out such as using your forearm and elbow to increase pressure while performing the massage.

You may even use your feet by standing or walking on your lover's back. However, these are not recommended if you are doing the massage in bed as the support the receiver's body has may not be firm. Explore these variations with your lover's consent. Another variation is to kiss and suck on your lover's toes or kiss behind the ears or suck on the earlobes.

Do so before applying any oil for the massage for obvious hygiene reasons. Also make sure your lover's feet are clean. We indicated in the beginning taking a bath or shower before the massage. You may also use a wet towel or dip the towel in some warm water to wet it and wipe your lover's body before the massage.

Turn over a new feel

Once you have finished massaging the back of your lover's head and neck, it's time to devote your attention to the front of your lover's body. Ask them to turn over and if you happen to see a strangely serene look or smile on your lover's face, then you can silently feel encouraged that you have succeeded so far in giving an enjoyable intimate massage.

Start with the feet as you did earlier and slowly progress up the legs. Be gentle and careful with the shin and the knees so as not to exert too much pressure on the bones whereas the front of the thighs can be kneaded with vigor. When you reach the groin, remember to tease sensually enough but refrain from indulging in any overt sexual stimulation. You can massage all around the sex centers and softly caress them to tease but do not rub vigorously your lover's vagina or stroke his genitals.

At this point, it is important to note that you may be tempted to indulge in a Yoni massage or a Lingam massage but refrain from doing so. As we mentioned earlier, the ideal time to perform a Yoni massage or a Lingam massage is after you complete the full body massage.

Of course, you may perform either the Yoni massage or Lingam massage on its own, as well. However abandoning a full-body massage halfway through and diverting your focus on either a Yoni or Lingam massage will disrupt the flow and disturb the benefits of relaxation gained so far.

When you massage the lower abdomen and stomach, be careful not to exert too much pressure. Following this, you will enjoy the next phase of massaging your lover's chest region. It is important to be gentle when you are massaging female breasts whereas the male chest can withstand more pressure. Use soft circular strokes and caresses on the female breasts but you can knead and even tap the male chest.

Pinching and rubbing both the female and male nipples and the flesh around them are allowed. However, ask your lover's feedback if you see them flinch or grimace when you do so. Kissing the breasts or chest and sucking on the nipples are variations you may practice after seeking consent.

After this, sit facing your lover's head and massage their shoulders, neck, head, face and forehead. Be careful when you massage the neck not to exert too much pressure on the front of the neck but evenly on the sides. Ideally stroke, rub or caress the neck and face.

Similarly, be very careful when you massage the face not to poke your fingers in the eyes. In fact, for heightened sensuality, you may place a piece of cloth on his or her eyes or blindfold your lover. This is entirely optional and subject to mutual agreement. Kissing is optional and as always with the receiver's consent.

End the massage with long, soft and slow strokes and caresses on your lover's forehead starting from the middle and going towards both sides.

Congratulations. You have completed a full body intimate massage and it is now time to receive feedback.

Communicate

An ideal way to communicate is for the massage giver to lie down and join his or her lover for a cuddle. Use a blanket or sheet to cover yourself if you wish to. Once you have found comfort in each other's body warmth, the giver may initiate the communication by asking questions if there was anything he or she did wrong or if the receiver would prefer to make any changes to the ritual.

It is important for the receiver to be honest in providing feedback so that the massage giver can improve his or her technique the next time. For instance, if the receiver felt the giver could devote more time to a certain part of the body during the massage, she or he should say so. Or the receiver can also say something like you can be more bold or firm with my thighs or my breasts.

The receiver can also compliment the giver if she or he enjoyed any particular technique or aspect of the massage. You can also plan and discuss any changes that you may wish to integrate into the massage for the next session.

Now that you know the technique, you may be keen to try it out. However, there are a few more important aspects to consider including some interesting massage techniques such as the Yoni massage to give her pleasure and the Lingam massage to give him pleasure which we will explain and you can explore in the subsequent chapters.

So, let's now look at some preparatory steps to create the right environment or ambience for an intimate and sensual full body massage.

Setting the Mood

Creating the right environment and mood for an intimate massage is as important as the massage itself. Being disturbed halfway through the massage or finding out that you are feeling cold or uncomfortable can spoil the experience.

An abandoned or interrupted intimate massage can have long-term effects on you and put you off from trying it again because you are afraid of being disappointed again. It is therefore important that you take the following preparatory steps to ensure you and your lover enjoy a complete, blissful and fulfilling massage session.

Peace and privacy

Make sure that you will be undisturbed during the massage. This means planning and preparing to eliminate any potential interruptions. The last thing you want is to receive a phone call during the massage. So turn off your phone or put it in silent mode. Make sure the place or room is quiet, peaceful and pleasant, and that it also affords privacy. Lock the door and put a 'Do Not Disturb' sign if you are in a hotel room. If you are at home, then choose a time that is appropriate when it will be less likely to expect friends or family to come visiting.

The stereotypical ambience will mean closing the windows and drawing the blinds or curtain closed, dimming the lights and playing some soft music. However, there are no hard and fast rules to do so. You can leave the windows open or the curtains open, if you want to and think that you will still have privacy. You may also prefer silence instead of playing any music.

The lights are also optional. You may dim them or keep them as usual. Some people prefer to light candles or some incense. Talk it over with your lover and choose what you both prefer and feel comfortable with.

Set the temperature on the air conditioner before you begin. Remember that as the body relaxes, the receiver may tend to feel cold, so don't turn the thermostat too low or the fan too high. At the same time, if it is summer and you are in a place that has tropical weather, then be prepared to sweat. Keep some towels and a jug of cool lemonade or water with some glasses nearby and handy.

Feather the nest

More than music or lighting candles, the most important part of preparing for an intimate massage is to choose the place where the receiver will be comfortable. If you are willing to invest in a professional massage table, that's well and good but you don't necessarily have to.

You can lay a mat on the floor and place some clean sheets or a blanket for your lover to lie down. Though some people don't mind using the bed, it's not ideal nor comfortable for various reasons. For instance, you will be using oil during the massage which may stain the mattress. Another very valid reason is that the surface of the bed is not as firm as the floor and this is important for the receiver's comfort.

Clear a place on the floor and arrange everything required; a mat or a thin mattress, some sheets, some blankets, cushions or pillows, towels, oil and anything else you may need.

It's up to you to lubricate or not

Using oil as a lubricant during the massage is optional. Some people may prefer not to use any oil. Not using oil for a full body massage is permissible but it is recommended that you use some kind of lubricant to perform the Yoni massage or the Lingam massage. Since both these massages involve contact with highly sensitive parts such as the vagina, clitoris, penis or testicles, not using oil or lubricant can cause discomfort or even pain.

If you are using oil, then make sure it is suitable for massage. Some of the most commonly preferred massage oils are almond oil, coconut oil or grapeseed oil.

Use oil that is natural and or organic rather than something that is synthetically concocted or blended. It is also a good idea to use oils that you have tried and tested. You don't want any skin irritation, rashes or any form allergic reaction.

Bathe or shower

It is recommended that you bathe or shower before a massage to truly enjoy it. It is also healthy and hygienic to do so. A nice slow warm bath before beginning your massage will help relax the muscles and also make the skin feel supple. You may also consider taking a shower together before beginning to set the mood for intimacy.

An intimate massage session has the power to take you to heights of pleasure you've never before experienced. So prepare well to enjoy the pleasure without any limitations or hiccups. In the next two chapters, we look at some of the most intimate ways to pleasure your lover.

These techniques may seem like foreplay because they involve direct contact and massage of your lover's erogenous zones and sexual parts but it is essential to keep in mind that you don't necessarily need to have a goal of sexual intercourse or orgasm.

These intensely pleasurable massage techniques will enable you to experience intense erotic sensations if you are willing to explore them for their own sake and without any prejudice or preconceived expectations. These massages can help you connect not just physically and sexually but emotionally and spiritually as well.

Give Her Pleasure (Yoni Massage)

In ancient Tantric traditions, the physical body is considered as sacred and the genitals are given particular importance as marking the location of one of the centers of energy, also known as chakra. The base chakra or energy center in the human body is believed to be located within and around the area of the genitals.

This is the reason why a woman's vagina (or a man's penis for that matter) is always referred to with respect. Thus the Sanskrit word for the vagina, which is Yoni, is used with reverence and does not in any way have any derogatory or negative connotation the way the terms, pussy, twat, cunt or even vagina, have in English.

Yoni massage is a form of worship

In fact, many interpretations of the word, Yoni, attribute its meaning as signifying a 'sacred place' or 'temple.' Therefore, it is important that both the giver and the receiver approach the Yoni massage technique that we describe here as a form of worship. There should be no shame, or any other negative feelings associated with the massage.

While the benefits of the massage may apparently seem to be physical and sexual in nature, it is more than just erotic foreplay. In Tantric traditions, the Yoni massage is considered to be spiritually and emotionally empowering as it is sexually and physically beneficial.

According to Tantra, a Yoni massage can help clear any blockage of energy in a woman's base chakra, increase blood flow in the sexual organs and aid in expelling toxins from the body. By stimulating the energy center, it allows the life force or 'Prana' to flow freely within the woman's body, thus promoting general health and wellbeing in the receiver.

On an erotic level, it provides unprecedented pleasure to the receiver by encouraging them to shed their inhibitions and embrace new ways of exploring their sensual potential. New and intense sensations are just the tip of the iceberg. By giving your lover a Yoni massage, you are opening the doors to a whole new way of making an erotic as well as an emotional and spiritual connection.

Expect the extremely ecstatic

Before we begin, it is important to note that the Yoni massage may or may not lead to the receiver experiencing an orgasm. However, this should not be the goal or focus of the massage. It is an expression of deep love and devotion from the giver to the receiver.

Enjoy the massage slowly and do not hurry. Do not worry about the outcome but instead allocate a specific time, preferably an hour or more, for the massage. Remember that unlike a man, the woman's body needs anywhere between half an hour to an hour to be fully aroused and stimulated.

The first time a person receives the Yoni massage, it can be a very powerful and intense experience. It can be emotionally overwhelming and expressing what you feel as freely as possible is important.

Moaning, sighing, crying out loudly or breaking into sobs or tears are not just allowed but encouraged as they are an indication of the receiver's erotic pleasure as well as emotional release and cleansing. They also compliment the devotion and prowess with which the receiver is giving the Yoni massage. At any point during the massage, the receiver can make any suggestions or indicate that she does not want to continue, if she so choses.

Prepare to worship

As part of the preparation for a Yoni massage session, it is important that the giver and receiver cleanse themselves to avoid any chances of infection. Taking a bath or shower and washing thoroughly the genitals (especially the receiver's), the hands and fingers (especially the giver's), and under the nails are important. A misplaced sense of hygiene associates the genitals with being dirty. Therefore, ensuring that the receiver has no inhibitions, shame or guilt in exposing her vagina and the receiver in touching it is important.

Empty your bladders just before you begin, so you do not get uncomfortable during the massage. Shaving the receiver's pubic hair is recommended as smoothly shaven genitals can significantly increase the receiver's sensitivity and pleasure. A well-oiled vagina is also a pleasure to behold for both the giver and receiver and a clean-shaven vagina without any pubic hairs will enhance your visual pleasure.

Similarly, trimming the massage giver's fingernails is recommended to avoid any irritation caused by scratching. However, these are optional and a matter of preference. Use organic, natural and pure oil or a water-based lubricant. Using the right lubricant or oil is absolutely necessary as the vagina is extremely sensitive and any irritation can spoil the pleasure potential of a Yoni massage.

The receiver can choose to be completely naked or just naked from the waist below. Similarly the giver can choose to be completely naked or half naked from the waist above or even fully clothed.

Position yourself for maximum pleasure

The receiver has the right to choose where she wants to receive the Yoni Massage. Unlike a full body massage, you can perform the Yoni massage on a firm bed or mattress if you wish to. Just be careful not to spill or drip any oil or lubricant. It makes sense to use layers of bath towels or some extra sheets to cover the bed to soak up any oil or lubricant that may seep or flow from the receiver's body.

Alternatively, the receiver may choose to receive the Yoni massage lying down on a mat or mattress on the floor. You may use a professional massage table, if you have one. Make sure there is enough room for both the receiver to lie down and the giver to either sit or stand. One of the most comfortable and conventional positions for the receiver to enjoy a Yoni massage is for her to lie on her back with her legs spread apart and bent at the knees.

Place one or two pillows or cushions so that her upper body can be inclined at an angle from where she can comfortably have a view of the receiver's hands on her Yoni or vagina. This is so that the receiver can have visual pleasure as well as sensory pleasure.

Alternatively, the receiver may choose to lie down so that her upper body is flat on the floor, massage table or bed. In this position, she may also choose to place a blindfold on her eyes, as this can contribute to sharpening her sensory feelings.

The massage giver will sit cross-legged on the floor or bed between the receiver's legs. If you are using a massage table, then the giver may stand at the end of the table or sit or stand beside it whichever position gives a comfortable way to reach with the hands between the receiver's legs.

There are variations for the receiver's position to choose according to comfort and preference which we shall explore towards the end of the chapter. It is also a good idea to try out different positions during subsequent massage sessions to experiment with your comfort and the intensity of your sensations.

Hold heaven in your hands

Start by warming your hands (this is addressed to the massage giver) by rubbing them together. Use your hands to gently caress your lover's inner thighs and lower belly. Maintain eye contact with the receiver if she finds it comfortable. Try various movements with your hands and fingers such as tapping with the palm or drumming with your fingertips. The receiver may communicate which movement she prefers.

Do this for a few minutes without touching her Yoni or vagina but gently teasing all around it. You are trying to stimulate blood circulation and awaken the skin and flesh to every slight sensory experience. The idea is to allow the receiver to completely relax and release any tension that her body feels.

Pay attention to her breathing so that you can sense the quickening or shallowing of her breath as she gets excited or relaxes. It is important to take long, deep breaths so that the receiver is able to completely relax and enjoy the Yoni massage.

When you sense that she is ready, ask her permission to place your palm on her vagina. Put your palm facing down on her vaginal mound complete covering it. You should realize that this is a significant movement. You are in a sense holding heaven in your hands because both of you should feel a sense of blissful connection with each other.

Give her pleasure in four ways

There are four main techniques or parts involved in the Yoni massage. We'll describe each of them below. Of course, there are other variations that you will learn to try on your own as you start practicing the massage regularly. In Tantric tradition, it is recommended that you use your right hand to massage the Yoni or vagina. You may use both hands to increase the intensity or vary the rhythm of the massage.

Massaging the labia

Keep your palm face down covering the vaginal mound for a while and feel the warmth. Then slowly start caressing her Yoni or rubbing your palm over her vaginal mound. Apply some oil or lubricant and continue to caress all around and on the vagina.

After a while slowly trail the middle finger along the crease of the vaginal opening between her labia or the lips on either side of her vagina. Use long and gentle upward and downward strokes to stimulate the vagina.

These movements will increase blood flow in the region and allow her Yoni to swell and open. Continue stroking the vagina externally for as long as you feel comfortable. The pleasure the receiver feels is extremely exquisite and by doing it for just the right amount of time builds up the expectation for what will come later.

Use the fingers on either side of the middle finger to slowly spread her labia. While continuing to massage her labia, use your middle finger to gently caress and stimulate the clitoris with each upward and downward stroke. Do not insert your finger into her vagina yet.

Massaging the clitoris

Slowly trail your thumb upward along the vaginal opening till you reach the clitoris. Use your thumb to gently rub the clitoris in a steady up and down rhythm, as if ringing a doorbell. Make sure you use enough oil or lubricant to keep your movements smooth. After a while, use your thumb to gently rub the clitoris in sideways motions.

Next, use your index finger to rub the clitoris in circular motions, clockwise and then anti clockwise. Spend some time rubbing the clitoris in every direction on an imaginary compass or marking every hour on an imaginary clock. You may also use your thumb and forefinger to gently pinch or squeeze the clitoris after seeking the receiver's permission.

Stroking the clitoris can awaken a whole new world of sensory experience for the receiver since it has more nerve endings than any other part of the body. Continue to stroke the clitoris as long as you both feel comfortable or until the receiver indicates you to stop.

Massaging the vagina

Insert your middle finger inside the vagina with your palm facing upward. Slowly, move your fingers in and out of her vagina. Start slow and then build up a steady or vigorous rhythm. Alternate or vary your rhythms to prolong her pleasure. The receiver can indicate a preferred rhythm of movement or give instructions to the giver by saying to go slow or to go fast.

After a while, seek the receiver's permission to insert two fingers, the middle and the ring fingers, and then continue the rhythmic vaginal massage. Vary your movements by massaging the inside walls of her vagina, imagining a compass and your fingers going north, north east, east and so on in a clockwise and then in an anti-clockwise direction.

While massaging the vagina, seek the receiver's permission to massage her perineum. This is the area between her vagina and anus and is a particularly sensitive and erogenous zone.

If you are feeling adventurous, then you may insert your little finger or pinky in her anus, after seeking her permission. Continuing to gently stroke her anus, vagina or Yoni and clitoris at the same time can be an intensely pleasurable experience for the receiver.

On a light-hearted Tantric note, it is said that when you have your pinky in her anus, your ring and middle fingers in her Yoni or vagina and your thumb on her clitoris, then your index finger is pointing towards the meaning of life.

Massaging the G-spot

Insert your middle finger inside her vagina and curl or hook it as in a come-hither gesture. The idea is to use your finger to stimulate her G-spot, which is located an inch or so inside the vagina on the upper wall. The receiver can guide the giver to move his finger in the right direction if she feels necessary. Use the tip of your middle finger to gently massage the G-spot.

The Yoni may produce nectar.

Remember, achieving an orgasm is not necessary but if you do, then go with the flow of your body. Some first time massage receivers have been known to experience multiple orgasms or an orgasm that may last for a pretty long while. The receiver can choose to continue the massage following an orgasm or even while having an orgasm.

While having an orgasm or during the massage, the receiver may feel like she needs to urinate. This feeling of the need to urinate can actually be a feeling that she needs to ejaculate and it can be easily confused.

The female ejaculate is a clear liquid unlike the male ejaculate and therefore can be easily mistaken for urine. However, the ejaculate is discharged from the prostate gland and not the urethra. In Tantric traditions, this ejaculate is considered very sacred and referred to as the nectar of life.

The giver and receiver may by mutual consent also agree not to have an orgasm but use the Yoni massage to prolong the pleasurable sensations for as long as possible. This means playing a cat and mouse game of pleasing and teasing so that the receiver's pleasure peaks and then falls.

The giver will help the receiver to reach a state of sensation where she is almost going to have an orgasm and then stop or slow down the rhythm to help her to relax. This will need excellent communication and coordination between the lovers and can also be immensely satisfying in helping the receiver to relax and the giver to explore her desires.

Concluding the massage gradually and not abruptly is essential. Use your palm to cover her vaginal mound towards the end of the session and feel the warmth emanating from her body. You may hold her hand with your other hand while doing so, if she is comfortable.

Following the massage, lying down together for a cuddle or hugging each other will allow you to talk about it. If she prefers to lie down silently, that's also fine.

Experiment with positions

Instead of lying facing up with her legs spread wide and knees bent, the receiver may explore different positions. The main intentions are to be comfortable and also to maximize the sensation of pleasure. The receiver may lie face down with a cushion or a rolled up towel placed under her groin and hips to raise them. Another variation is to lie flat on her back with her knees tucked into her chest and one hand holding around the back of her knees with her legs high up in the air. In any of these positions, it is necessary to allow maximum exposure of the receiver's Yoni so that it is comfortably accessible for massage and stimulation by the giver's hands.

She may also lie sideways. For instance, she may lie on her right side with her right leg stretched straight and her left leg bent at the knee. This will allow the giver to sit by her side, facing her legs and use both hands to massage her Yoni.

Another variation that you can explore is for the receiver to sit on an armchair with her knees spread and legs dangling from the arms of the chair. She may also kneel on the armchair with her hands on the back of the chair.

Finally, some tips and advice. Bring an open mind. Leave behind your inhibitions. Remember that the Yoni massage is all about the giver giving the receiver pleasure. Needless, to say, the giver of the massage can be a man or a woman.

The receiver can also have two people give her a massage simultaneously. One of them can devote his or her attention to her upper body or breasts while the other focusses on her Yoni or vagina. This can be an intensely erotic experience for the receiver. It is up to the receiver or the couple to mutually decide to either have two male or two female or one male and one female massage givers, according to preference.

It is important to note that there is nothing expected from the receiver in return. In Tantric tradition, the Yoni massage is a ritual offering by the massage giver to the receiver. The massage giver is expected to treat the receiver of the massage just like a deity or goddess, in a religious ritual, with love and reverence. The giver should keep the sanctity of the massage intact by not expecting a Lingam massage in return or initiating intercourse following the massage.

Giving a woman a Yoni massage is a gift of love and devotion. A man (or woman) by giving a woman a Yoni massage not only intensifies her pleasure but strengthens their relationship on multiple levels, emotional as well as sexual.

In our next chapter we look at the Lingam massage where the massage giver devotes attention on giving him pleasure. Ideally the Lingam massage should not be connected to the Yoni massage or performed as if in exchange for the Yoni massage.

It is recommended that a Yoni massage and a Lingam massage are performed on separate days so that the receiver and the giver have the pleasure of enjoying and devoting their time for each session wholeheartedly.

Give Him Pleasure (Lingam Massage)

While the term Lingam in Sanskrit, refers only to the penis, the Lingam massage may involve massaging more than just the penis. The massage can be extended to include the testicles, the perineum and the prostate.

In Tantric tradition, the Lingam massage is likened to a ritual worship of the male phallus symbolizing the creative energy of the universe. According to Tantric theories, the root chakra or energy center that houses the life force is located at the base of the spine.

Performing a Lingam massage is believed to awaken the Kundalini or primal energy which is lying coiled within a man. This energy is not only sexual or libidinal but also associated with intuitive instincts and spiritual awareness.

A man receiving the lingam massage will therefore not only benefit from a feeling of being sexually invigorated but also contribute to restoring his emotional equilibrium. By performing a Lingam massage for your lover, you will be able to help him overcome any negative emotions, as well as improve his confidence.

Surrender your will

The objective of a Lingam massage is not to enable the receiver to achieve orgasm but to prolong his pleasure and take him to edge as many times as possible. An orgasm may be how the Lingam massage culminates or it may not. In Tantric tradition, when the giver performs the Lingam massage to allow the receiver to repeatedly feel erotic pleasure but prevents ejaculation, it is intended to improve his virility and physical stamina. It can at the same time heighten his erotic sensation and capacity for pleasure as well.

A couple may mutually agree or the receiver may choose not to orgasm during the Lingam massage. However, whether the Lingam massage leads to an orgasm or not is secondary. The primary objective of the Lingam massage is to help the receiver relax and passively receive the sensations of pleasure.

Traditionally, men are expected to take control and this leads to the expression of aggression in their actions. The Lingam massage provides an opportunity for a man to let go of his masculine ego and get in touch with the softer and gentler aspects of his personality.

For the Lingam massage to work effectively, the receiver needs to surrender. He needs to let go of goal-oriented, active behavior and passively repose his trust in the massage giver's hands, literally.

Take the lead

The giver takes the lead in preparing the receiver for the Lingam massage. Since men conventionally think that the pressure to perform or play an active role in a relationship is expected of them, they need to relax and let go of any such leadership notions and allow the giver to take control of the Lingam massage session.

Prepare for the Lingam massage by thoroughly cleansing yourself and your lover. Taking a bath or shower together is a good idea. Otherwise, take turns to wash the entire body. Pay special attention to the genitals and hands.

Shaving the male genitals is recommended to enhance the receiver's sensory pleasure and the giver's visual joy. However, this is purely a matter of preference. It is also recommended that the massage giver ensures nails on their hands are cut or trimmed before the massage.

The giver and the receiver of the Lingam massage may choose to be completely naked during the massage. On the other hand, the receiver may choose to be naked from the waist down and the giver may choose to be naked from the waist up or even fully clothed.

You may perform the massage on a bed or on a mat placed on the floor, or even a massage table if you have one. Make sure that you place towels or sheets to soak up any oil or lubricant that may flow from the receiver's body when you are performing the massage.

Being worried about causing stains on the mattress or spilling oil or lubricant should be the last thing on your mind. Complete focus is important for both the receiver to relax and the giver to devote attention to the massage.

Once you have cleansed your bodies, the giver of the massage leads the receiver to the place where the massage is to be performed. This ritual signifies the receiver relinquishing control and placing his trust in the giver's hands. To make it interesting and symbolic, the receiver may choose to be blindfolded. The giver may hold the receiver's Lingam or penis and lead him to the massage table, bed or a mat on the floor.

This marks a new equation where the giver of the Lingam massage plays an active role and the receiver a passive role until the massage session is over.

Put him in place before you begin

The conventional position is for the receiver to lie flat on his back on a mat on the floor, the bed or the massage table. His legs are spread apart at an angle that is comfortable. The massage giver may choose to kneel or sit cross-legged between his legs or sit beside him whichever is comfortable. If the massage is performed on a massage table, then obviously the giver will stand on the side of the table.

Begin by rubbing together your hands (this is addressed to the giver). Then gently tap and drum your fingers on the inside of his thighs and lower abdomen. After a while, gently caress or massage all around his genitals without touching either the penis or testicles.

Pay careful attention to your breathing as well as his breathing. It is important that you use this preparatory massage period to enable him to relax. Remember to take long deep breaths. At times of excitement, breathing can become shallow and remembering to breathe deep will enhance your enjoyment of the massage. This applies to both the giver and the receiver of the massage.

Play with pleasure in three ways

There are three parts to the Lingam massage where the giver pays attention to the receiver's testicles, his penis or Lingam and his perineum in a progressive fashion. We will describe below some standard massage techniques or movements for each part.

Feel free to modify or improvise these techniques. The penis is pretty supple and strong, and can withstand some amount of pulling, twisting and pressing. It is important that the receiver communicate to the giver when his pain threshold is crossed or if any action or technique causes discomfort.

Perform the massage akin to a ritual in an orderly fashion while keeping in mind that an orgasm or ejaculation is not the goal. During each part of the massage or in-between applying a movement or technique, take a few minutes' break to allow the receiver to relax if he gets too aroused or excited.

It is alright if the penis goes flaccid or alternates between becoming erect and then going soft. In fact, some techniques work better when the penis is soft and flaccid. So time your movements to allow the blood flow in the genital area to recede and enable the receiver to relax.

Massaging the testicles

Pour oil or lubricant on your hands or apply some drops on his testicles. Start by gently scooping the testicles from below in your left hand. Hold them in your hand by encircling your lover's testicles with your thumb and forefinger at the base where it hangs from below the penis.

Hold this position for a while and use your right hand to gently massage the testicles with your fingers and the palm alternately. Ask the receiver's permission to gently squeeze with your left hand at the base or tug at the testicles.

If the penis becomes erect, hold still for a while and let it relax. Then continue massaging the testicles. Depending on whether you are right-handed or left-handed, you can choose to hold with either the right or the left hand and similarly use the other hand to massage.

Massaging the penis

While still holding the testicles in one hand, encircle his penis with your other hand and slowly glide your hand from the base of the penis up towards the head and then back down, in long gentle strokes.

Stop if you feel that the receiver is nearing ejaculation allowing him to relax. The receiver may also indicate if he wants the giver to slow down the rhythm or stop for a while. Massaging the perineum at regular intervals will help the receiver relax and also allow him to control ejaculation. After performing these strokes, move on to the next technique of twisting the penis. Let go of the testicles and use both hands to encircle the penis. Depending on the length of the penis, you may use all your fingers on both hands to encircle or just a few of them.

Now twist each hand in opposite directions. The penis may be erect or go soft, as you loosen and tighten your grip. Continue twisting while holding a loose grip so that it creates friction and a slightly tighter grip as if gently wringing the penis. Next, hold the penis in between both palms while keeping your palm and fingers straight. Now start moving your hands in opposite directions. The movement is similar to rubbing your palms together but with your lover's penis in between. This movement is believed to raise the energy that is lying dormant within the base chakra.

In the next technique, hold the penis by encircling it in one hand and then pulling, tugging or bending it in all different directions or towards each hour of an imaginary clock. Perform this movement clockwise and then anticlockwise.

After a few strokes, follow this movement by encircling just below the head of the penis with your thumb and forefinger. Then move one hand in ten upward motions followed by ten downward motions. Use the other hand and repeat and then use both hands alternately.

Do not worry if the penis goes soft or ejaculates. You can continue the massage unless the receiver requests you to stop. Keep a towel handy in case you wish to wipe the ejaculate.

Massaging the perineum

Make your hand into a fist and gently push it against the perineum which is located between the testicles and the anus. Gently massage using your knuckles. You can alternate by using your thumb to massage the perineum.

Massaging the perineum is an excellent way to help the receiver relax and lose the urge to ejaculate. You can use this technique repeatedly while massaging the penis to allow the penis to grow soft whenever you want to.

If the receiver and the giver mutually agree, then you can experiment with the prostate massage. This involves the massage giver inserting the index finger in the receiver's anus palm facing upwards and crooking the finger.

About an inch inside the anus and towards the front of the male body is the prostate. Massaging the prostate with a finger curved in a come-hither gesture is considered by some as the male equivalent of massaging the female G-spot.

Please note that many heterosexual men may not be comfortable and may even feel violated by the prostate massage. It is therefore important to discuss and agree in advance whether to include it in your Lingam massage or not.

End happily

In contrast to the conventional happy ending that most men seek during a massage, the Lingam massage may not necessarily end in ejaculation. A couple may mutually agree to try and deliberately avoid ejaculation. This requires a good level of coordination and communication between the giver and receiver.

Contrary to popular belief, not ejaculating does not necessarily mean not achieving an orgasm. According to some ancient traditions, regularly not ejaculating for a while will also help the receiver to improve his libido and sexual stamina. However, this is a matter of choice and comfort. A couple may discuss the potential outcome and mutually agree according to whatever they find pleasurable and relaxing.

Another alternative way to end the massage is to time it. So set an alarm to go off, half an hour later or after however long you want the massage to last. This does not mean that the giver abruptly stops the massage when the alarm goes off. Instead the alarm is an indication to the couple to slowly begin winding down and prepare to end the Lingam massage in the next 10 minutes or so.

Following the end of the massage, the massage giver can lie down and cuddle or hold hands with the receiver.

Do's and Don'ts

The words 'intimate massage' usually bring to mind sexual foreplay or free and uninhibited behavior. This is generally true but as we have seen, some order of ritual needs to be followed and some knowledge of techniques can go a long way in enhancing the pleasure you derive from an intimate massage session.

In the same manner, there are some dos and don'ts which can clearly prevent misunderstandings or discomfort during an intimate massage session. While these dos and don'ts may not seem as important or exciting as the technique, they however play an integral role in ensuring your pleasure.

Do's for the massage giver:

- Do prepare the place by getting all the necessary items such as towels, sheets, cushions, oil or lubricant etc.
- Do turn off the phones, lock the door and prepare for any potential disturbances.
- Do set the mood and the ambience by playing music or dimming the lights or lighting some incense.
- Do choose the right oil or lubricant after consulting with the receiver.
- Do warm up the oil if required after checking with the receiver.
- Do ask for feedback at regular intervals from your lover to ensure he or she is comfortable and enjoying the massage.
- Do vary your strokes, rhythm, speed and technique by including as much variety as possible.
- Do enjoy giving the massage because it can contribute to your lover's pleasure.

Don'ts for the massage giver:

- Don't hurry the massage session because the whole point is to help your lover relax and rushing through it can be counter-productive.
- Don't pour or splash oil directly on your lover's body as it may cause discomfort. Instead pour some on your hands and apply or gently dab a drop or two on your lover's body.
- Don't use your thumbs too much because it can tire you out too soon and too easily. Instead vary your techniques often by using all your fingers, different parts of your palms and hands and in different ways.
- Don't use the bed if you can use the floor or a massage table. The bed rarely provides a firm surface which is ideal for massage and may often cause discomfort to your lover.
- Don't use too much force or pressure and hurt your lover.
- Don't wear a wristwatch, rings, bangles, bracelets or other jewelry which may interfere with the massage.
- Don't do it if you don't enjoy it. It is pointless and will only harm the relationship.
- Don't take advantage of your lover by trying out something new without discussing beforehand or without seeking permission.
- Do not expect a massage in return. The last thing your lover wants to hear following a massage is, "Okay, now it's my turn." Ideally, the receiver should not perform massage on the same day that he or she receives one.

Do's for the receiver

- Do provide feedback to guide and encourage the massage giver.
- Do relax and be comfortable otherwise you will make the massage giver nervous.
- Do indicate if you feel any pain or discomfort at any point during the massage or from any particular technique of massage.

Don'ts for the receiver

- Don't try to take control of the massage by micro-managing the massage giver's actions or constantly giving instructions. Allow the giver to do his or her job but do give feedback occasionally.
- Don't grin and bear pain or discomfort. People have different levels of sensitivity and your response will help the giver apply the right pressure and use the appropriate techniques.
- Don't hold in your emotions. A massage is a means to relax physically as well as emotionally and mentally. Sighing or moaning are allowed and may even be considered a compliment by the giver.

The Importance of Communication

In spite of all the necessary preparations, a couple may not be able to enjoy a massage completely if they do not communicate before, after and during the massage. An intimate massage is an opportunity for lovers to communicate and connect on a physical, intellectual, emotional and even spiritual level. And communication is the key to connecting with your lover.

Before the massage: Set any ground rules before beginning the massage. Discuss why you want to do the intimate massage and mutually agree that it is something you both want and are comfortable doing.

During the massage: If there are any specific parts of the body or techniques that you wish to avoid, say so. In BDSM sex, participants use what is called a safe word to stop when the submissive feels the pain or discomfort is unbearable. Similarly, agree on a code using hand signals or movement of the head to communicate or provide feedback. Just saying it aloud is easy but sometimes talking may seem like it takes too much effort when you are in a relaxed mood while receiving the massage.

So lifting up your index finger may mean your answer is yes and lifting two fingers, your index finger and middle finger may mean no. Similarly a thumbs-up sign may indicate your enjoyment and mean giving encouragement to the massage giver to go on. A raised hand palm open may indicate you wish the giver to stop doing what he or she is doing.

After the massage: Spend some time going over the techniques and express your feelings following the massage session while you are cuddling or holding hands. Talk about your feelings while they are still fresh in your mind.

Any kind of feedback that will contribute to improve the next massage session is welcome.

Also be generous with your compliments. Irrespective of whether you received or gave a massage, express your enjoyment. It will encourage your lover to be more relaxed or more confident during the next massage session.

THE END

"TANTRIC Massage: THE BEGINNER'S GUIDE"   by Dominique Atkinson

Introduction

Let's imagine that you've just won a prize. Maybe you participated in the company raffle or accidentally clicked some online promotion. Perhaps there were forms involved, or online surveys that were filled out or maybe a friend entered your name into a draw.

The "hows" and "whys" are up to you; what's important is that you've won. Now, suppose the winning envelope arrives in the mail, and at first you're skeptical. It's natural. Little in life is free, and it's likely that someone's just trying to get you to buy into something, pay a deposit, or offer up your credit card information. Scams and fraud are everywhere these days, but this worry evaporates as you read the letter inside the envelope.

You've really won! It's completely free, and there are no strings attached! But that's not what surprises you the most. What you've just won is a free Tantric massage. Just imagine how you'd react. Envision what it is you've won. Is there some secret spa, hidden in the heart of the city, which you need to visit? Or is there a phone number for you to call, to arrange for home service? When the moment arrives, are there fragrant oils in the air? Does your masseuse light candles in the background?

Now, picture the masseuse. Are you being massaged by a man or a woman? Are they clothed or naked? Is this masseuse young or old? Do you chat away like old friends or does your masseuse maintain a more professional attitude? What about the massage itself? Do you imagine it as intense as a deep-tissue massage? Or does your mind conjure a progression of light touches, as sensual as they are stimulating? Do you expect the experience to completely blow your mind?

If you've never experienced a Tantric massage, your imagination can only take you so far. You're probably struggling to answer a simple question; What exactly is a Tantric massage?

What Is Tantric Massage?

Most people will agree there's something sensual and seductive, even outright sexual, about the act of Tantric massage. Thanks to popular culture, even those who've never experienced one know that there's something erotic and pleasurable about the act.

This is hardly surprising, as the word "Tantra" is generally understood to have sexual connotations. Taking this into consideration, it's logical to assume that a Tantric massage is either a highly sexual activity or serves as an introduction to one.

You may even know of someone who's tried it, or you've seen one of the many advertisements out there (usually at health spas that also offer full body massages, aromatherapy, or acupressure). It's even possible that you've tried out one of these services, and your experience has helped you understand what Tantric massage really is.

The Definition of Tantric Massage

The basic definition of Tantric massage is that it's a form of sensual massage that makes use of Tantric practices to achieve relaxation and a sense of calm. Unlike some forms of massage, Tantric massage may involve touching or stimulating the genitals in order to achieve greater pleasure and relaxation. This massage is also considered a spiritual practice, one that can help both the masseuse and their subject attain a greater understanding of the world.

This definition matches with classic Tantric practices and generally works well under the framework of Neotantra. But how do we define the secular forms of Tantric massage, those missing the elements of spirituality introduced by Tantra? Would a Tantric massage, performed by someone who doesn't practice Tantra, be only an erotic or sexual massage?

Some Tantric practitioners believe that massages performed without the spiritual elements of Tantra aren't true Tantric massages. This is understandable; the very name implies the incorporation of Tantric elements, and they should be present in a form beyond mere emulation. For those new to Tantric massage, however, identifying and staying true to these spiritual elements may prove difficult.

Other Tantric practitioners believe that it is possible to perform a Tantric massage without the spiritual elements. They argue that the end result would still be a form of Tantric massage, but they concede that it wouldn't have the full impact that a Tantric massage would otherwise have, when performed by a Tantric practitioner.

Part of this rationale involves one of the key principles of Tantra that states that all experiences can be used to achieve enlightenment or knowledge of the divine. If we accept this, what might be perceived as an inferior form of Tantric massage, as practiced by one with no concern for spirituality, could still lead to a spiritual experience.

On the other hand, there are people who don't believe in the spiritual benefits of Tantric massage. They believe it can be practiced to full effect by using principles that don't rely on the elements of Tantra. It's their opinion that the techniques, methods, and skill of the masseuse are enough to achieve the full effect of a Tantric massage.

The Parable of the Elephant and the Blind Men

Which of these definitions and beliefs are correct? Perhaps part of the answer can be found in the parable of the elephant and the blind men.

One day, six blind men found themselves trying to define what an elephant is. They each reached out towards the elephant and described what it was they could feel.

One blind man touched the elephant's leg and said, "An elephant is like a pillar!"

Another blind man gripped the elephant's tail and said, "No, an elephant is like a strong rope!"

The third blind man ran his hands along the elephant's trunk and said, "I believe an elephant is like the branch of a tree!"

The fourth stroked the elephant's ear and said, "Actually, an elephant is like a large fan!"

The fifth felt the stomach of the elephant and said, "No, no. An elephant is like a wall!"

The last blind man touched the tusks of the elephant and said, "You are all fools! An elephant is like a spear!"

The blind men continued to argue over the definition of the elephant until someone who could see came upon them and explained that they each held a different part of the elephant. It took someone who could see the whole picture to tell them they were all correct, and that they were all mistaken.

Clearly, each blind man made a truthful observation based on what they'd experienced. But since none of them were able to experience the entire elephant, they're unable to describe the elephant as a whole.

In one sense of the parable, we can understand that the various descriptions and beliefs concerning Tantric massage come from the fact that each person's experience of it is different, perhaps imperfect or selective. It could be said that some of these descriptions reflect only a certain part of the elephant, or an amalgam of several parts at most.

Another point to take away from this parable is that it took a man with sight, one who could observe the bigger picture, to reveal to the blind men that all their differing opinions were part and parcel to something much bigger than they were able to realize. It was only through the sharing of this knowledge that the blind men were able to come to a greater understanding of the world around them.

So, what is Tantric massage? As the parable suggests, perhaps the answer lies in a combination of all the unique views people have of it, and that enlightenment may come from being able to see the bigger picture this book hopes to reveal.

A Brief Introduction to Tantra

Tantric massage is derived from the traditions of Tantra. Acquiring a basic understanding of Tantra is one of the first steps towards a better understanding of Tantric massage itself.

Despite how familiar the word has become through pop culture hype, Tantra is still widely misunderstood by the general public. This is especially true in the western world, where it's mistakenly perceived that Tantra is all about sex, a myth popularized by a focus on the practice of Tantric sex. This localized, mainstream interest in Tantra is at least partly why Tantric massage remains misunderstood today.

Let's clear it up now. Despite what most people know, Tantra is actually a collection of spiritual beliefs and rituals that were originally developed in India over a thousand years ago. While it is not a religion itself, it's managed to influence established religions through its beliefs and practices. One of its central tenets was to work towards achieving a heightened sense spirituality and enlightenment, and the acts of Tantric sex and Tantric massage are simply the most well-known methods of this, two methods out of a diverse repertoire of rituals belonging to Tantra.

A Brief History of Tantra

Tantra is believed to have originated from the rituals of small tribal communities in East India anywhere from 100 to 300 C.E., although the oldest writings on Tantra are thought to have been transcribed around 500 C.E. By this time, the scattered rituals of these tribal communities had come together to form a more unified and more detailed tradition.

Tantra has always been an esoteric system of belief from its inception, a tradition of secrecy that only permitted the teachings to be passed down from a master, or guru, to a student worthy of the knowledge. Regardless, this didn't prevent its teachings from influencing every major religion in India over the passing centuries. It spread through the country alongside Hindu and Buddhist beliefs, and even influenced the practice of Islam in some areas.

As Hinduism gained popularity in India, Buddhism moved east and took the practice of Tantra with it. It eventually reached the Indo-China subcontinent, influencing even the Japanese practice of Buddhism.

In the twentieth century, a growing interest in the religions and philosophies of the East resulted in the western discovery of Tantra. Brought to North America along with Hindu and Buddhist spiritual beliefs, Tantra eventually merged with New Age philosophies and spirituality. This form of Tantra eventually became better known as Neotantra. This "new Tantra" combines western thought and philosophy with the practices of Tantra, maintaining many of Tantra's core beliefs.

Today's practice of Tantric massage comes mostly from the teachings of Neotantra, although some do claim to have been taught Hindu or Buddhist Tantric traditions. Less concerned with secrecy, the practice of Neotantra has allowed more people to become aware of at least a few traditional Tantric practices. Inevitably, there are some who believe this to be a corruption of Tantra, but there are others who believe that it may well be the modern take on an ancient path to spirituality.

Basic Tantric Beliefs

It would be wrong to think that Tantra is a single, cohesive, and coherent system of beliefs. As Tantra was originally taught only from guru to student, different forms began to develop over the centuries, as certain gurus stressed certain teachings or passed along revelations that differed from other Tantric practitioners.

Despite its relative infancy, or perhaps even because of it, not even the practice of Neotantra can be considered a cohesive whole. Teachers of various forms of Neotantra often maintained the basic, core beliefs of Tantra, but just as often had differing beliefs in certain areas and specific practices.

That being said, there are still a number of common beliefs shared by most, if not all the different forms of Tantra.

Goals of Tantra

The common goal of many styles of Tantra is to achieve a greater understanding of the universe through understanding the self as it experiences life. It's believed that the practice of Tantra elevates even the most mundane and normal experiences, allowing enlightenment to come from things as simple as enjoying a delicious meal to something as dynamic as the act of sex.

This materialistic philosophy contrasts with other approaches to spirituality, whose followers often seek to separate themselves from worldly things and experiences. Instead of denying the world, Tantra embraces it, and at times it even encourages the methodical breaking of perceived taboos, such as the use of alcohol or hallucinogens, or the practice of sacred sexuality. These acts are not meant to be done for their own sake; rather, practitioners believed that, by breaking taboos, one could achieve a greater awareness of the world and the universe.

Energy, or Prana

Tantric practitioners believe in the existence of energy, or *prana,* which flows through the universe, including the bodies of practitioners. Many rituals and practices of Tantra include the harnessing and use of *prana* in order to achieve spiritual and material goals. Meditation and breathing exercises are used in order to effectively channel *prana*, and some practices also involve the use of visualization exercises similar to the one in this book's introduction.

More relevant to the practice of Tantric massage, Tantra believes that there are two forms of energy in the body: masculine and feminine. These two forms of energy oppose each other but are also complementary, comprising two parts of a whole. Depending on the Tantric tradition, they are called "yang and yin" or "Shiva and Shakti".

Tantric massage manipulates and redirects the flow of these two energies within the receiver's body, with the giver of the massage functioning as the agent of this change. This allows Tantric massage to positively influence the body, mind, and spirit, allowing for improved physical and sexual health, focus, relaxation, and enlightenment.

The Importance of Personal Experience

Tantra believes that each person's experiences, and the ways in which these experiences may lead to enlightenment and wisdom, are unique to each individual. This is part of the reason why Tantra teaches how to achieve enlightenment, instead of instructing people on what enlightenment is. It simply cannot be taught, as the attainment of enlightenment is closely linked to a person's unique journey towards it.

In relation to the practice of Tantric massage, this means that each massage is not only intimate and sensual, but also highly personal and unique. The basic principles and techniques of the massage remain the same and are used as the means to achieve growth and spiritual enlightenment, but the experience can vary depending on both the giver and the receiver of the massage.

Tantra, or Not Tantra?

There's some debate about whether or not Neotantra, and thus the practice of Tantric massage, can even be considered a Tantric practice at all. While many forms of Neotantra remain true to the spirituality of Tantra, some forms are more secular and exist outside of spiritual practice, borrowing only the physical techniques and methods of Tantra.

Some argue that Neotantric practices that are divorced from Tantric spirituality should not be considered a Tantric form at all, since Tantra, from its inception, was concerned with man's spiritual quest to understand both the divine and the universe around them. Others believe that this may simply be a more modern approach to Tantra, one that is more relevant to the time and culture that spawned it.

In the end, this debate may be another variation of the parable of the elephant and the blind men, where one's comprehension is limited by their point of view. There may come a time when it is realized that truth may require a combination of ideas from many people who currently disagree with each other. Time will tell, but for now, there are many who accept the practice of both Neotantra and Tantric massage.

Tantra and Tantric Massage

It should be clear by now that there are diverse opinions concerning the purpose and spiritual methods of Tantric massage. There are many who advocate a clear and almost inseparable link between Tantra and Tantric massage. On the other hand, there are those that believe that it's possible to separate the physical practice from its more spiritual origins.

Despite their differing opinions, both sides of the debate will generally agree that a grasp of the traditional roots of Tantra, and how they subsequently apply to Tantric massage, can be helpful to both the giver and the receiver in understanding the true depth of the experience of the massage itself.

Here are some of the most significant Tantric elements that apply to Tantric massage.

Chakras

Tantric tradition believes that there are seven main centers of spiritual energy in the human body. These main centers, called chakras, line up from the base of the spine to the top of the head, in a line that divides the body into two equal halves. Chakras not only collect spiritual energy but also help to direct its flow. Tantric practices often involve affecting these chakras, to help redirect or balance the flow of energy, which can help the body heal itself and improve certain mental functions such as focus, concentration, and creativity.

Each chakra has a unique role in the body, but the aim of Tantric massage is typically the sacral chakra, located in the pelvic area. The sacral chakra is essentially the pleasure center of the body and is responsible for emotions, sensuality, and our relationships with other people. Aside from this, the sacral chakra is also believed to be the center of human creativity.

Sexual Energy

Kundalini energy, also referred to as "sexual energy", is said to reside near either the sacral chakra or at the root chakra, located at the base of the spine. It is considered dormant until awakened, which can happen during sexual activity. Kundalini is then believed to rise up through the spine towards the brain as sexual feelings are aroused and stimulated, after which the energy turns around and proceeds towards the genitals, seeking release through orgasm.

Kundalini energy is considered to be responsible for more than just a person's orgasm, however. The term itself can be translated as "coiled snake," which can give the image of the kundalini as a powerful, dangerous form of energy just waiting to be unleashed. That energy is said to be able to power a person's enlightenment, a creative force that can lead to positive transformation and change. Conversely, it can also cause great chaos to a person in mind or body.

Tantric massage usually focuses its efforts on activating kundalini energy, or at least preparing the receiver for its awakening. Yet, even in this there are differing opinions: the first being that orgasm should not be achieved during the massage, in order to preserve and empower the kundalini, and the second stating that the kundalini will be frustrated if orgasm is not achieved.

Lingam and Yoni

One Tantric tradition that has made its way into the practice of Tantric massage is the use of the terms "Lingam" and "Yoni." These are the Sanskrit terms for "penis" and "vulva" respectively, used to convey a greater sense of respect and even love between participants in a Tantric massage. Love and respect are seen as important in Tantra, especially between lovers and spouses, and that applies to the practice of Tantric massage as well. It is especially important to emphasize this level of respect in today's culture, where the genitals are often treated and referred to in a disrespectful manner.

Aside from inspiring respect and love within the participants, both terms have a spiritual relevance in the practice of Tantra. A man's lingam is a representation of Shiva, a Hindu deity that also embodies masculine energy. A woman's yoni is a representation of Shakti, consort of Shiva, who is the personification of feminine energy. By using these terms, one can reinforce the significance of the masculine and feminine energies that are at work within the practice of Tantra.

Meditation and Breathing

Practitioners of Tantric massage often make use of meditation and breathing exercises, a method commonly used in Tantra. This grants both the masseuse and their subject more control over their breathing and allows them to focus during a massage. Examples of these meditation and breathing exercises will be given in a later chapter.

Benefits of Tantric Massage

People may have different reasons for receiving a Tantric massage, but many of those reasons benefit the receiver alone. Givers also benefit from the massage, but the ways are not often equivalent. This inequality is at least partly by design, as the giver in a Tantric massage is typically assumed to be the more experienced and knowledgeable participant, and can provide a more skillfully executed massage, from which the less experienced receiver can learn.

Here are some of the benefits you can receive from a Tantric massage.

- *Tantric massage can improve your breathing.* Both the receiver and giver of a Tantric massage are expected to keep their breathing even throughout the massage. Breathing exercises to practice this are usually recommended, but even the act of Tantric massage itself can lead to deeper, more consistent breathing. This in turn contributes to greater health, as the body's ability to take in oxygen increases. Improved breathing can also result in greater alertness and focus, as well as improving one's ability to relax.

- *Tantric massage can help you relax both body and mind.* Like other forms of massage, a Tantric massage can be used to relax both body and mind. Some people may even find the lighter touch of the Tantric massage to be effective in this. To ensure these levels of comfort, both participants are encouraged to communicate with each other, to voice their concerns and preferences even before the session begins. This can reassure the receiver that this is a safe place in which to relax and allows the giver to better understand their subject's needs as well.

- *Tantric massage helps to balance and harness your kundalini energy.* Kundalini energy is a potent form of spiritual energy that can be tapped into through Tantric massage. As discussed in the previous chapter, it can usually be activated through sexual stimulation, and can result in heightened sexual desire or even whole-body orgasm. It can also help bring about feelings of bliss and connectivity, as it enables the mind of the receiver to become more spiritually open. Essentially, it is believed that it is kundalini energy that most effectively allows a person to experience the divine during a Tantric massage.

- *Tantric massage can be used to create sexual arousal.* Tantric massage is often a way to encourage intimacy between couples, sexual arousal being the result of a mutual need to express this intimacy. This is brought about not only through the physical manipulation of the lingam or yoni, but also from the awakening of kundalini energy.

It should be noted that if you are receiving a massage from a professional masseuse, you should make the masseuse aware if you begin to feel sensations that make you uncomfortable. This will allow the masseuse to change their approach, or even stop if necessary.

- *Tantric massage can help one overcome sexual trauma.* This is a more recent application of Tantric massage, and one that is usually performed by a masseuse who is also a well-trained therapist. It is believed that a well-trained therapist can create a psychological and spiritual safe space for the receiver while performing the massage. In this way, the therapist is able to help the receiver along their healing journey. This practice should only be undertaken with great care, and only with a therapist that understands the boundaries that must be set for this to be done successfully.

- *Tantric massage can be a learning experience.* This reason is perhaps the closest to Tantric belief. One of the fundamental beliefs of Tantra is that even the most mundane experiences can allow a person to have a greater understanding of both themselves and the world around them. Through the combination of light and other stimuli, sensual massage aided by Tantric techniques, the receiver is given the opportunity to explore their inner selves, and the reality that surrounds them. On a less metaphysical level, receiving a Tantric massage can also expose you to new techniques and methods, which can then be used and practiced when your roles are reversed.

Made in the USA
Coppell, TX
31 January 2025

45147747R00026